BLOOD TYPE A+ DIET COOKBOOK

50+ Delicious Recipes for Your Blood Type to Achieve Optimal Health and Wellness

Copyright © 2024 by ADAM KABBANI

All rights reserved

This copyrights page explains the legal rights and protections related to the content of this nonfiction book for readers and users. You understand that you have the right to access or use this book in any way, including reading, downloading, or sharing. Ownership and Intellectual Property Rights: The content, graphics, and other elements in this nonfiction book are all covered by copyright and other intellectual property laws. Adam Kabbani is the only owner of the content. Any unauthorized use or reproduction of this book's content may be illegal and give rise to legal action. For reading and using this book for personal, non-commercial uses only, you have been granted a constrained, non-exclusive, and non-transferable permission. You are prohibited from altering, distributing or Without Adam Kabbani's prior written approval, you may not distribute, communicate, display, perform, reproduce, publish, license, create derivative works from, transfer, or sell any portion of the book

TABLE OF CONTENTS

Chapter 1: The Basics of Blood Type A+ Diet................. 1

Overview of Blood Type A+ Characteristics

Dietary Recommendations for Blood Type A+

Foods to Enjoy

Foods to Avoid

Chapter 2: Nutritional Needs for Blood Type A+....... 13

Essential Nutrients for Blood Type A+

Supplements and Vitamins

Hydration Tips

Chapter 3: Understanding Food Groups for Blood Type A+..17

Proteins for Blood Type A+

Fruits and Vegetables for Blood Type A+

Grains and Legumes for Blood Type A+

Dairy and Alternatives for Blood Type A+

Chapter 4: Recipes for Blood Type A+..........................26

Breakfast Ideas

Lunch Recipes

Dinner Recipes

Dessert Recipes

Chapter 5 : Meal Planning for Blood Type A+...........42

Creating Balanced Meals

Sample Meal Plans

Grocery Shopping Tips

Cooking Techniques for Blood Type A+

INTRODUCTION

Welcome to the Blood Type A+ Cookbook! This culinary guide is designed specifically for individuals with Blood Type A+ who are looking to optimize their health and well-being through a diet tailored to their genetic makeup.

The Blood Type Diet, popularized by Dr. Peter J. D'Adamo, suggests that our blood type influences how our bodies react to certain foods. According to this theory, individuals with Blood Type A+ may benefit from a diet rich in plant-based foods, lean proteins, and whole grains, while minimizing or avoiding certain animal proteins and processed foods.

In this cookbook, you'll find a diverse collection of delicious and nutritious recipes carefully crafted to support the dietary preferences of Blood Type A+

individuals. Whether you're new to the Blood Type Diet

or a seasoned practitioner looking for fresh culinary

inspiration, this cookbook aims to make meal planning

and cooking enjoyable and satisfying.

Each recipe in this cookbook is thoughtfully curated to

align with the nutritional recommendations for Blood

Type A+. From hearty breakfast options and vibrant

salads to comforting soups and flavorful main dishes,

you'll discover a variety of dishes to suit your taste

preferences and dietary needs.

Throughout this cookbook, you'll also find helpful tips

on ingredient substitutions, cooking techniques, and

meal planning strategies to support your journey

towards optimal health. Additionally, we've included a

comprehensive food list specific to Blood Type A+ to

guide you in making informed choices while grocery shopping and meal prepping.

We believe that eating well should never mean sacrificing flavor or enjoyment, and our goal with this cookbook is to empower you to embrace a nourishing and fulfilling culinary lifestyle that supports your unique blood type.

So, without further ado, let's embark on a delicious journey tailored to the needs of Blood Type A+ individuals. Get ready to savor the flavors, nourish your body, and thrive with the Blood Type A+ Cookbook as your culinary companion.

UNDERSTANDING BLOOD TYPE A+

Understanding Blood Type A+ is essential for tailoring dietary and lifestyle choices to optimize health and well-being. Blood Type A+ individuals have specific genetic markers on their red blood cells that distinguish them from other blood types. These individuals are believed to have descended from ancestors who primarily consumed an agrarian or agricultural diet.

In the context of the Blood Type Diet, individuals with Blood Type A+ are often described as having a sensitive immune system and a tendency towards heightened stress responses. As such, dietary recommendations typically emphasize a predominantly plant-based diet rich in fresh fruits, vegetables, legumes, and whole grains. Lean proteins such as fish and poultry are often preferred over red meat, which is suggested to be less compatible with the Blood Type A+ physiology.

Understanding Blood Type A+ also involves recognizing potential health implications and considerations. Research suggests that individuals with Blood Type A+ may have a higher susceptibility to certain health conditions, such as cardiovascular disease and cancer, and may benefit from targeted dietary and lifestyle interventions to mitigate these risks.

Overall, gaining a deeper understanding of Blood Type A+ enables individuals to make informed choices that align with their genetic predispositions, promoting optimal health and vitality. By embracing a diet and lifestyle tailored to their blood type, individuals with Blood Type A+ can optimize their overall well-being and potentially reduce the risk of developing chronic health conditions.

HOW THE BLOOD TYPE DIET WORKS

The Blood Type A+ diet is based on the premise that an individual's blood type influences how their body responds to certain foods. According to this theory, those with Blood Type A+ are believed to thrive on a primarily plant-based diet, resembling the dietary patterns of their agrarian ancestors.

The diet works by categorizing foods into three main groups: beneficial, neutral, and avoid. Beneficial foods are those believed to enhance health and well-being for Blood Type A+ individuals, while neutral foods are considered generally safe but may not offer specific benefits. Foods to avoid are those deemed incompatible with the Blood Type A+ physiology and are thought to potentially lead to health issues.

The diet's proponents claim that by adhering to these guidelines, individuals with Blood Type A+ can optimize their digestion, energy levels, and overall health. It is believed that consuming foods aligned with one's blood type can support proper metabolic function, reduce inflammation, and improve nutrient absorption.

Furthermore, the Blood Type A+ diet emphasizes the importance of lifestyle factors such as stress management and exercise in conjunction with dietary choices. By following this tailored approach, proponents suggest that individuals with Blood Type A+ can achieve better health outcomes and potentially reduce the risk of certain diseases. However, it's important to note that scientific evidence supporting the Blood Type Diet's efficacy is limited, and individual responses to the diet may vary.

BENEFITS OF EATING ACCORDING TO YOUR BLOOD TYPE

Eating according to your blood type, such as Blood Type A+, is purported to offer several potential benefits based on the principles of the Blood Type Diet. Proponents of this approach claim that aligning your diet with your blood type can lead to improved overall health and well-being.

One of the main benefits touted by the Blood Type Diet is enhanced digestion and nutrient absorption. By consuming foods that are deemed compatible with your blood type, it is believed that you can optimize your digestive processes and better absorb essential nutrients, leading to improved energy levels and overall vitality.

Proponents suggest that eating according to your blood type can support weight management efforts. By following a diet tailored to your genetic predispositions, you may be more likely to make food choices that promote satiety, regulate metabolism, and maintain a healthy weight.

Another purported benefit is improved immune function and reduced inflammation. The Blood Type Diet recommends certain foods that are believed to support the immune system and minimize inflammatory responses in the body, potentially reducing the risk of chronic diseases and promoting overall longevity.

Adherents of the Blood Type Diet often report experiencing increased energy levels, mental clarity, and overall well-being when following the dietary guidelines specific to their blood type.

While these benefits are frequently cited by proponents of the Blood Type Diet, it's important to note that scientific evidence supporting these claims is limited, and individual responses to the diet may vary. It's advisable to consult with a healthcare professional before making significant dietary changes based on blood type recommendations.

CHAPTER 1

THE BASICS OF BLOOD TYPE A+ DIET

The basics of the Blood Type A+ diet revolve around

tailoring dietary choices to align with the specific

genetic characteristics associated with Blood Type A+.

This diet is based on the concept that individuals with

Blood Type A+ may benefit from a predominantly plant-

based eating pattern, reminiscent of the agrarian

lifestyle of their ancestors.

Key principles of the Blood Type A+ diet include

consuming a variety of fresh fruits, vegetables, legumes,

and whole grains, while minimizing or avoiding certain

animal proteins and processed foods. Lean proteins

such as fish and poultry are often recommended over

red meat, which is believed to be less compatible with the Blood Type A+ physiology.

The diet categorizes foods into three main groups: beneficial, neutral, and avoid. Beneficial foods are those believed to support health and well-being for Blood Type A+ individuals, while avoid foods are considered less compatible and may potentially lead to health issues.

By adhering to the dietary recommendations of the Blood Type A+ diet, proponents suggest that individuals can optimize their digestion, energy levels, and overall health. However, it's important to note that scientific evidence supporting the efficacy of the Blood Type Diet is limited, and individual responses to the diet may vary.

OVERVIEW OF BLOOD TYPE A+ CHARACTERISTICS

Blood Type A+ is one of the four blood types determined by the presence or absence of specific antigens on the surface of red blood cells. Individuals with Blood Type A+ have both the A antigen and the Rh antigen, making them compatible with receiving blood transfusions from donors with Blood Types A or O and Rh+.

From a health perspective, those with Blood Type A+ are often described as having certain characteristic traits. They are believed to possess a strong immune system with a tendency towards heightened stress responses. This may result in a predisposition towards conditions such as heart disease, cancer, and autoimmune disorders. Consequently, individuals with Blood Type A+ are often encouraged to adopt dietary and lifestyle practices that support immune health and stress management.

In terms of personality traits, individuals with Blood Type A+ are often associated with being conscientious, detail-oriented, and organized. They may also be sensitive to environmental stimuli and have a preference for routine and structure in their daily lives.

While these characteristics are not deterministic and can vary widely among individuals, understanding the general tendencies associated with Blood Type A+ can provide insights into potential health considerations and inform personalized approaches to diet, lifestyle, and overall well-being.

DIETARY RECOMMENDATIONS FOR BLOOD TYPE A+

Dietary recommendations for Blood Type A+ individuals focus on consuming a predominantly plant-based diet with an emphasis on fresh fruits, vegetables, legumes, and whole grains. Lean proteins such as fish and poultry are typically preferred over red meat, which is believed to be less compatible with the Blood Type A+ physiology. Additionally, dairy products are often limited or avoided altogether, as they may cause digestive issues for some individuals with Blood Type A+.

Furthermore, individuals with Blood Type A+ are encouraged to prioritize organic and locally sourced foods whenever possible and to avoid processed and artificial ingredients. The diet also emphasizes the importance of mindful eating practices, such as chewing food thoroughly and eating in a relaxed environment.

By following these dietary recommendations,

individuals with Blood Type A+ aim to support optimal

health and well-being tailored to their genetic

predispositions.

FOODS TO ENJOY

Understanding your unique blood type can provide

valuable insights into the foods that best support your

health and vitality Foods to Enjoy for Blood Type A+:

1. Leafy Greens: Incorporate nutrient-rich leafy greens

such as kale, spinach, and Swiss chard into your meals.

These greens are packed with vitamins, minerals, and

antioxidants that support overall health.

2. Soy Products: Tofu, tempeh, and edamame are

excellent sources of plant-based protein for Blood Type

A+ individuals. Choose organic, non-GMO soy products to reap their nutritional benefits.

3. Berries: Enjoy a variety of berries such as blueberries, strawberries, and raspberries, which are rich in antioxidants and vitamins. These colorful fruits can be enjoyed fresh or added to smoothies and desserts.

4. Legumes: Incorporate legumes like lentils, chickpeas, and black beans into your meals for a healthy dose of protein, fiber, and essential nutrients. These versatile ingredients are great additions to soups, salads, and main dishes.

5. Whole Grains: Opt for whole grains such as quinoa, brown rice, and barley, which provide sustained energy and are rich in fiber and minerals. These grains can be used as bases for meals or enjoyed as side dishes.

6. Vegetables: Fill your plate with a variety of colorful vegetables, including broccoli, carrots, and bell peppers. These vegetables are low in calories and high in vitamins, minerals, and antioxidants, supporting overall health and well-being.

7. Fish: Incorporate fatty fish like salmon, mackerel, and trout into your diet for a healthy source of omega-3 fatty acids and protein. Aim to include fish in your meals a few times per week for optimal health benefits.

8. Green Tea: Enjoy a cup of green tea as a refreshing and antioxidant-rich beverage. Green tea is known for its health-promoting properties and can be enjoyed hot or cold throughout the day.

Adding these nutritious foods into your diet, you can support your Blood Type A+ physiology and enhance your overall health and well-being. Experiment with different recipes and meal combinations to enjoy a diverse and satisfying diet that aligns with your blood type.

FOODS TO AVOID

Understanding which foods to include and which to avoid is key to supporting your well-being on this journey.

1. Red Meat: Beef, lamb, and pork are commonly recommended to be avoided or minimized for individuals with Blood Type A+ due to their potential negative impact on digestion and metabolism.

2. Dairy: Dairy products, including milk, cheese, and yogurt, may be challenging for some Blood Type A+ individuals to digest efficiently and are thus often suggested to be limited or substituted with alternatives.

3. Wheat: Foods containing wheat, such as bread, pasta, and baked goods, are often discouraged for Blood Type A+ individuals, as they are believed to contribute to inflammation and digestive issues.

4. Corn: Corn and corn-derived products are considered less compatible with the Blood Type A+ physiology and may be best avoided or consumed in moderation.

5. Processed and Fried Foods: Highly processed and fried foods, including fast food items and snacks, are generally not recommended for Blood Type A+

individuals due to their low nutritional value and potential adverse effects on health.

6. Shellfish: Certain types of shellfish, such as shrimp, crab, and lobster, are often advised to be limited or avoided by Blood Type A+ individuals due to potential allergic reactions or digestive discomfort.

7. Kidney Beans: While legumes are generally recommended for Blood Type A+ individuals, kidney beans are an exception and are often suggested to be avoided due to their lectin content, which may interfere with digestion.

8. Peanuts and Peanut Butter: Peanuts and peanut-derived products are typically advised to be avoided or minimized for Blood Type A+ individuals due to their

lectin content and potential adverse effects on

digestion and immune function.

By being mindful of these foods to avoid and making

informed dietary choices, individuals with Blood Type

A+ can better support their overall health and well-

being in alignment with their genetic predispositions.

CHAPTER 2

NUTRITIONAL NEEDS FOR BLOOD TYPE A+

ESSENTIAL NUTRIENTS FOR BLOOD TYPE A+

Essential nutrients play a crucial role in supporting the health and well-being of individuals with Blood Type A+. While dietary recommendations may vary based on individual needs and preferences, certain nutrients are particularly important for optimizing health in this blood type group.

1. Vitamin A: Found in foods like carrots, sweet potatoes, and spinach, vitamin A supports immune function and vision health for Blood Type A+ individuals.

2. Vitamin C: Abundant in citrus fruits, bell peppers, and broccoli, vitamin C promotes collagen formation and enhances immune function, vital for overall health.

3. Folate: Essential for DNA synthesis and cell division, folate is found in leafy greens, lentils, and avocado, supporting cardiovascular and nervous system health.

4. Iron: Leafy greens, lentils, and tofu are rich sources of iron, crucial for oxygen transport and energy production in Blood Type A+ individuals.

5. Omega-3 Fatty Acids: Found in fatty fish like salmon, flaxseeds, and walnuts, omega-3 fatty acids support heart health and reduce inflammation, benefiting overall well-being for Blood Type A+.

Ensuring adequate intake of these essential nutrients through a well-balanced diet is key to supporting optimal health and vitality for individuals with Blood Type A+.

Supplements and vitamins can play a complementary role in supporting the nutritional needs of individuals with Blood Type A+. While a balanced diet is crucial, certain supplements may address specific deficiencies or enhance overall well-being. Blood Type A+ individuals may benefit from supplements such as vitamin B12, which is primarily found in animal products that are limited in this diet, as well as vitamin D, omega-3 fatty acids, and probiotics to support immune health and digestion. However, it's essential to consult with a healthcare professional or registered dietitian before starting any new supplement regimen, as individual needs may vary. Additionally, incorporating whole foods rich in these nutrients whenever possible is encouraged to optimize nutrient absorption and promote overall health.

HYDRATION TIPS

Proper hydration is essential for overall health, and individuals with Blood Type A+ can optimize their hydration routine with a few key tips. Firstly, aim to drink plenty of water throughout the day, as it supports digestion, nutrient absorption, and overall bodily functions. Herbal teas, especially those with soothing properties like chamomile or peppermint, can also contribute to hydration. Coconut water is another hydrating option that aligns well with the Blood Type A+ diet, providing electrolytes and minerals. It's advisable to limit or avoid sugary and caffeinated beverages, as they can lead to dehydration and may not be well-tolerated by some Blood Type A+ individuals. Lastly, listen to your body's thirst cues and adjust your fluid

intake accordingly to maintain optimal hydration levels.

CHAPTER 3

UNDERSTANDING FOOD GROUPS FOR BLOOD TYPE A+

Understanding food groups for Blood Type A+ involves

categorizing foods based on their compatibility with this

blood type's physiology. Beneficial foods for Blood Type

A+ include fresh fruits, vegetables, legumes, and whole

grains, which are believed to support optimal health

and digestion. Lean proteins such as fish and poultry are

also encouraged, while red meat and certain dairy

products may be limited.

Fruits and vegetables rich in antioxidants and fiber play

a crucial role in supporting the immune system and

promoting gut health for Blood Type A+ individuals.

Whole grains provide essential nutrients and sustained energy without causing digestive discomfort. Additionally, incorporating plant-based proteins like legumes ensures adequate protein intake while minimizing reliance on animal-derived sources.

By understanding and incorporating these food groups into their diet, individuals with Blood Type A+ can optimize their nutrition and support their overall well-being.

PROTEINS FOR BLOOD TYPE A+

Proteins play a crucial role in the diet of Blood Type A+ individuals, providing essential nutrients for optimal health. Here are five protein sources recommended for Blood Type A+:

1. Fish: Fish such as salmon, mackerel, and trout are rich in omega-3 fatty acids, which support heart health and cognitive function. These fatty acids also have anti-inflammatory properties, benefiting Blood Type A+ individuals who are prone to inflammation-related issues.

2. Poultry: Chicken and turkey are lean sources of protein for Blood Type A+ individuals. They provide essential amino acids necessary for muscle repair and growth without the saturated fat found in red meat.

3. Soy Products: Soy products like tofu, tempeh, and edamame are plant-based sources of protein suitable for Blood Type A+. They are also rich in phytoestrogens, which may have hormonal balancing effects beneficial for individuals with this blood type.

4. Legumes: Legumes such as lentils, chickpeas, and

black beans are excellent sources of plant-based protein

for Blood Type A+ individuals. They are also high in

fiber, aiding digestion and promoting satiety.

5. Nuts and Seeds: Almonds, walnuts, chia seeds, and

hemp seeds are nutrient-dense protein sources for

Blood Type A+. They provide healthy fats, vitamins, and

minerals, contributing to overall well-being.

FRUITS AND VEGETABLES FOR BLOOD TYPE A+

1. Berries (Beneficial): Berries such as blueberries,

strawberries, and raspberries are rich in antioxidants

and phytonutrients, which support immune function

and reduce inflammation. They are excellent choices for

Blood Type A+ individuals due to their potential health

benefits and compatibility with this blood type's

physiology.

2. Leafy Greens (Beneficial): Leafy greens like spinach,

kale, and Swiss chard are highly nutritious and rich in

vitamins, minerals, and fiber. They support digestive

health and provide essential nutrients such as vitamin K,

folate, and iron, making them beneficial options for

Blood Type A+ individuals.

3. Apples (Neutral): Apples are a versatile fruit that can

be enjoyed raw or cooked and are considered neutral

for Blood Type A+ individuals. While they may not offer

specific benefits, they are a good source of dietary fiber

and antioxidants, promoting overall health and well-

being when consumed in moderation.

4. Broccoli (Beneficial): Broccoli is a cruciferous vegetable rich in vitamins, minerals, and phytonutrients that support detoxification and immune function. It is a beneficial choice for Blood Type A+ individuals, offering a range of health benefits and supporting optimal health.

5. Sweet Potatoes (Beneficial): Sweet potatoes are a nutritious root vegetable rich in vitamins, minerals, and fiber. They have a lower glycemic index compared to regular potatoes and provide sustained energy without causing spikes in blood sugar levels. Blood Type A+ individuals can benefit from including sweet potatoes in their diet as a source of complex carbohydrates and essential nutrients.

Grains and Legumes for Blood Type A+

1. Amaranth: This gluten-free grain is considered

beneficial for Blood Type A+ individuals. It's rich in

protein, fiber, and various vitamins and minerals.

2. Oats: Whole oats are often recommended for Blood

Type A+ individuals. They provide soluble fiber, which

can help with digestion and cholesterol levels.

3. Rice: Brown rice is a staple in the Blood Type A+ diet.

It's easily digestible and provides energy without

causing spikes in blood sugar levels.

Legumes:

1. Lentils: Lentils are a great source of protein and fiber

for Blood Type A+ individuals. They're versatile and can

be used in various dishes like soups, stews, and salads.

2. Black-Eyed Peas: These legumes are considered beneficial for Blood Type A+ individuals. They're rich in fiber, folate, and other nutrients.

3. Soybeans (in moderation): Some Blood Type A+ individuals may tolerate soybeans well, but others may need to consume them in moderation. Soybeans are rich in protein and can be consumed as tofu, tempeh, or edamame.

Dairy and Alternatives for Blood Type A+

When considering dairy and alternatives for Blood Type A+ individuals, it's important to keep in mind that dairy products, particularly those high in fat and lactose, may not be well-tolerated by everyone with this blood type. Instead, individuals with Blood Type A+ may opt for

dairy alternatives that are easier to digest and less likely
to cause inflammation.

These alternatives typically include plant-based options
such as almond milk, coconut milk, oat milk, rice milk,
and soy milk (non-GMO). These alternatives offer
various nutritional benefits and can be used in place of
dairy milk in recipes or consumed on their own.

By incorporating these dairy alternatives into their diet,
Blood Type A+ individuals can ensure they are meeting
their nutritional needs while avoiding potential
discomfort associated with dairy consumption. It's
essential to experiment with different alternatives to
find the ones that best suit individual preferences and
dietary requirements.

RECIPES FOR BLOOD TYPE A+

Breakfast Ideas

1. Oatmeal with Fresh Fruit: Oats are a great source of fiber and complex carbohydrates, providing sustained energy throughout the morning. Fresh fruits add vitamins, minerals, and antioxidants for overall health.

2. Smoothie Bowl: Spinach is rich in iron and antioxidants, while bananas and berries provide natural sweetness and additional vitamins and minerals. Almond milk offers a dairy-free source of calcium and vitamin E.

3. Avocado Toast: Avocado is packed with healthy fats that help keep you feeling full and satisfied, while whole

grain toast provides fiber for digestive health. Tomatoes add vitamin C and antioxidants.

4. Greek Yogurt Parfait: Greek yogurt is high in protein, which helps support muscle repair and growth. Berries are rich in antioxidants, while granola adds crunch and fiber.

5. Quinoa Breakfast Bowl: Quinoa is a complete protein, containing all nine essential amino acids, making it an excellent choice for vegetarians or those looking to increase their protein intake. Sweet potatoes provide complex carbohydrates and beta-carotene.

6. Egg Muffins: Eggs are a great source of high-quality protein and essential nutrients like choline and vitamin D. Spinach and bell peppers add fiber and antioxidants.

7. Chia Seed Pudding: Chia seeds are rich in omega-3 fatty acids, fiber, and protein, making them a nutritious addition to any breakfast. Almond milk provides calcium and vitamin E, while fresh fruit adds natural sweetness and additional nutrients.

8. Tofu Scramble: Tofu is a plant-based source of protein and contains all essential amino acids. Spinach and bell peppers add fiber, vitamins, and minerals.

9. Whole Grain Pancakes: Whole grain flour provides complex carbohydrates and fiber, while bananas offer natural sweetness and potassium. Almond butter adds healthy fats and additional protein.

10. Breakfast Burrito: Eggs are a nutrient-dense source of protein and essential nutrients like vitamin B12 and

selenium. Black beans provide fiber and plant-based protein, while avocado adds healthy fats and fiber.

These breakfast ideas are not only delicious but also provide a balance of nutrients to support overall health and well-being for individuals with Blood Type A+.

Lunch

1. Salmon Salad: Grilled salmon served on a bed of mixed greens with cherry tomatoes, cucumber slices, and a lemon vinaigrette. Salmon is rich in omega-3 fatty acids, which support heart health and brain function.

2. Quinoa Salad: Quinoa mixed with diced bell peppers, cucumber, black beans, corn, and a cilantro lime dressing. Quinoa is a complete protein and a good source of fiber, while vegetables provide vitamins and minerals.

3. Turkey Wrap: Whole grain wrap filled with sliced turkey breast, avocado, lettuce, and tomato. Turkey is a lean source of protein, while avocado adds healthy fats and fiber.

4. Stir-Fried Tofu and Vegetables: Tofu stir-fried with broccoli, bell peppers, snap peas, and carrots in a ginger garlic sauce. Tofu is a plant-based source of protein, while vegetables provide fiber and essential nutrients.

5. Mediterranean Chickpea Salad: Chickpeas tossed with diced cucumber, tomatoes, red onion, olives, and feta cheese in a lemon herb dressing. Chickpeas are a good source of plant-based protein and fiber.

6. Lentil Soup: Hearty lentil soup made with lentils, carrots, celery, onions, and tomatoes. Lentils are rich in

protein, fiber, and essential nutrients like iron and folate.

7. Grilled Chicken Caesar Salad: Grilled chicken breast served on a bed of romaine lettuce with Caesar dressing, Parmesan cheese, and whole grain croutons. Chicken is a lean source of protein, while romaine lettuce provides vitamins and minerals.

8. Vegetable Sushi Rolls: Nori sheets filled with brown rice, avocado, cucumber, carrots, and bell peppers. Sushi rolls are low in calories and provide a good source of carbohydrates and fiber.

9. Chickpea Avocado Wrap: Whole grain wrap filled with mashed avocado, chickpeas, spinach, and diced tomatoes. Chickpeas are a good source of plant-based protein and fiber, while avocado adds healthy fats.

10. Vegetable and Bean Burrito Bowl: Brown rice

topped with black beans, sautéed bell peppers, onions,

corn, avocado slices, and salsa. Black beans are rich in

protein and fiber, while vegetables provide essential

nutrients.

These lunch ideas are not only nutritious and satisfying

but also aligned with the dietary recommendations for

individuals with Blood Type A+.

Dinner Recipes

1. Grilled Salmon with Roasted Vegetables: Grilled

salmon served with a side of roasted sweet potatoes,

Brussels sprouts, and carrots. Salmon is rich in omega-3

fatty acids, while vegetables provide vitamins, minerals,

and fiber.

2. Vegetable Stir-Fry with Tofu: Tofu stir-fried with broccoli, bell peppers, snap peas, carrots, and mushrooms in a ginger garlic sauce. Tofu is a plant-based source of protein, while vegetables provide essential nutrients and fiber.

3. Quinoa Stuffed Bell Peppers: Bell peppers stuffed with cooked quinoa, black beans, corn, diced tomatoes, and spices. Quinoa is a complete protein, while black beans provide additional protein and fiber.

4. Chicken and Vegetable Skewers: Grilled chicken skewers with bell peppers, onions, and zucchini. Chicken is a lean source of protein, while vegetables offer vitamins, minerals, and fiber.

5. Turkey and Spinach Meatballs: Turkey meatballs made with ground turkey, spinach, garlic, and herbs

served with marinara sauce over whole grain pasta.
Turkey is a lean source of protein, while spinach adds
vitamins and minerals.

6. Vegetable Curry with Chickpeas: Chickpea and
vegetable curry made with coconut milk, tomatoes,
curry powder, and spices served over brown rice.
Chickpeas are a good source of plant-based protein and
fiber.

7. Mushroom and Spinach Quinoa Risotto: Quinoa
cooked with mushrooms, spinach, onions, garlic, and
vegetable broth until creamy. Quinoa is a complete
protein, while mushrooms and spinach provide vitamins
and minerals.

8. Lentil and Vegetable Soup: Hearty lentil soup made
with lentils, carrots, celery, onions, tomatoes, and

spices. Lentils are rich in protein, fiber, and essential nutrients like iron and folate.

9. Baked Cod with Roasted Vegetables: Baked cod fillets served with a side of roasted asparagus, cherry tomatoes, and cauliflower. Cod is a lean source of protein, while vegetables offer vitamins, minerals, and fiber.

10. Chickpea and Spinach Coconut Curry: Chickpea and spinach curry cooked in coconut milk with onions, garlic, ginger, and spices served over brown rice. Chickpeas are a good source of plant-based protein and fiber, while spinach adds vitamins and minerals.

These dinner recipes are not only delicious and satisfying but also aligned with the dietary recommendations for individuals with Blood Type A+.

Snack Options

1. Greek Yogurt with Berries: Greek yogurt topped with

mixed berries such as strawberries, blueberries, and

raspberries. Greek yogurt is rich in protein and calcium,

while berries provide antioxidants and vitamins.

2. Almond Butter on Rice Cakes: Whole grain rice cakes

spread with almond butter. Almond butter is a good

source of healthy fats and protein, while rice cakes

provide carbohydrates and fiber.

3. Hummus and Vegetable Sticks: Hummus served with

sliced cucumbers, carrots, and bell peppers. Hummus is

made from chickpeas, which are a good source of plant-

based protein and fiber, while vegetables provide

essential nutrients and fiber.

4. Apple Slices with Almond Butter: Apple slices dipped in almond butter. Apples are rich in fiber and antioxidants, while almond butter adds healthy fats and protein.

5. Trail Mix: A mix of raw nuts such as almonds, walnuts, and cashews with dried fruits like apricots, raisins, and cranberries. Trail mix provides a balance of healthy fats, protein, and carbohydrates, as well as vitamins and minerals from the dried fruits.

6. Edamame: Steamed edamame sprinkled with sea salt. Edamame is a good source of plant-based protein and fiber, as well as vitamins and minerals like folate and vitamin K.

7. Greek Yogurt Parfait: Layer Greek yogurt with granola and mixed berries. Greek yogurt provides protein and

calcium, while granola adds crunch and fiber, and

berries provide antioxidants and vitamins.

8. Vegetable Sushi Rolls: Nori sheets filled with brown

rice, avocado, cucumber, carrots, and bell peppers.

Sushi rolls are low in calories and provide a good source

of carbohydrates and fiber, as well as vitamins and

minerals from the vegetables.

9. Roasted Chickpeas: Chickpeas seasoned with spices

like paprika, cumin, and garlic powder, then roasted

until crispy. Chickpeas are a good source of plant-based

protein and fiber, as well as vitamins and minerals.

10. Dark Chocolate Covered Almonds: Raw almonds

dipped in dark chocolate. Dark chocolate is rich in

antioxidants, while almonds provide healthy fats and

protein.

These snack ideas are not only delicious and satisfying but also aligned with the dietary recommendations for individuals with Blood Type A+.

Dessert Recipes

1. Fruit Salad with Honey-Lime Dressing: A refreshing mix of seasonal fruits such as strawberries, kiwi, pineapple, and grapes, drizzled with a honey-lime dressing. This dessert is naturally sweet and packed with vitamins, minerals, and antioxidants from the fruits.

2. Banana "Nice" Cream: Frozen bananas blended until creamy and smooth, then topped with chopped nuts or shredded coconut. This dessert is dairy-free, naturally sweetened, and provides potassium and fiber from the

bananas, along with healthy fats and protein from the nuts or coconut.

3. Chia Seed Pudding: Chia seeds soaked in almond milk with a touch of vanilla extract and sweetened with a natural sweetener like maple syrup or honey, then chilled until thickened. Chia seeds are rich in omega-3 fatty acids, fiber, and protein, making this dessert both nutritious and satisfying.

4. Baked Apples with Cinnamon: Apples cored and baked until tender, then sprinkled with cinnamon and served warm. This simple dessert is naturally sweet, low in calories, and provides fiber and antioxidants from the apples, along with blood sugar-regulating properties from the cinnamon.

5. Dark Chocolate-Covered Strawberries: Fresh strawberries dipped in melted dark chocolate and chilled until set. Dark chocolate is rich in antioxidants and may have heart-healthy benefits, while strawberries provide vitamins, minerals, and fiber.

6. Coconut Yogurt Parfait: Layers of dairy-free coconut yogurt, granola, and mixed berries in a glass. This dessert is dairy-free, gluten-free, and provides probiotics from the coconut yogurt, fiber and crunch from the granola, and vitamins and antioxidants from the berries.

These dessert recipes are not only delicious and satisfying but also aligned with the dietary recommendations for individuals with Blood Type A+.

MEAL PLANNING FOR BLOOD TYPE A+

Day 1:

- Breakfast: Oatmeal with Fresh Fruit (oats, banana, berries)

- Lunch: Greek Yogurt Parfait (Greek yogurt, mixed berries, granola)

- Dinner: Grilled Salmon with Roasted Vegetables (salmon, sweet potatoes, Brussels sprouts, carrots)

- Snack: Hummus and Vegetable Sticks (hummus, cucumber, carrots, bell peppers)

Day 2:

- Breakfast: Smoothie Bowl (spinach, banana, almond

milk, protein powder, granola, sliced almonds, fresh fruit)

- Lunch: Quinoa Salad (quinoa, bell peppers, cucumber, black beans, corn, cilantro lime dressing)

- Dinner: Vegetable Stir-Fry with Tofu (tofu, broccoli, bell peppers, snap peas, carrots, mushrooms, ginger garlic sauce)

- Snack: Apple Slices with Almond Butter (apple, almond butter)

Day 3:

- Breakfast: Avocado Toast (whole grain toast, mashed avocado, sliced tomatoes, pumpkin seeds)

- Lunch: Lentil and Vegetable Soup (lentils, carrots, celery, onions, tomatoes)

- Dinner: Turkey and Spinach Meatballs with Marinara Sauce over Whole Grain Pasta (ground turkey, spinach, garlic, herbs, marinara sauce, whole grain pasta)

- Snack: Trail Mix (almonds, walnuts, cashews, apricots, raisins, cranberries)

Day 4:

- Breakfast: Chia Seed Pudding (chia seeds, almond milk, vanilla extract, maple syrup)

- Lunch: Chickpea and Spinach Coconut Curry (chickpeas, spinach, coconut milk, onions, garlic, ginger, spices, brown rice)

- Dinner: Chicken and Vegetable Skewers (chicken, bell peppers, onions, zucchini)

- Snack: Roasted Chickpeas (chickpeas, paprika, cumin,

garlic powder)

Day 5:

- Breakfast: Vegetable Sushi Rolls (nori sheets, brown

rice, avocado, cucumber, carrots, bell peppers)

- Lunch: Mushroom and Spinach Quinoa Risotto

(quinoa, mushrooms, spinach, onions, garlic, vegetable

broth)

- Dinner: Baked Cod with Roasted Vegetables (cod,

asparagus, cherry tomatoes, cauliflower)

- Snack: Dark Chocolate Covered Almonds (dark

chocolate, almonds)

Day 6:

- Breakfast: Whole Grain Pancakes (whole grain flour, bananas, almond butter)

- Lunch: Mediterranean Chickpea Salad (chickpeas, cucumber, tomatoes, red onion, olives, feta cheese, lemon herb dressing)

- Dinner: Vegetable Curry with Chickpeas (chickpeas, coconut milk, tomatoes, curry powder, spices, brown rice)

- Snack: Edamame (steamed edamame, sea salt)

Day 7:

- Breakfast: Egg Muffins (eggs, spinach, bell peppers,

feta cheese)

- Lunch: Turkey Wrap (whole grain wrap, turkey breast,

avocado, lettuce, tomato)

- Dinner: Quinoa Stuffed Bell Peppers (bell peppers,

quinoa, black beans, corn, diced tomatoes, spices)

- Snack: Fruit Salad with Honey-Lime Dressing

(strawberries, kiwi, pineapple, grapes, honey-lime

dressing)

This meal plan provides a variety of nutritious and

delicious meals and snacks that are aligned with the

dietary recommendations for individuals with Blood

Type A+. Feel free to adjust portion sizes and

ingredients to suit individual preferences and dietary

needs.

CONCLUSION

The Blood Type A+ Diet Cookbook offers a comprehensive guide to optimizing health and well-being through personalized nutrition. By understanding the unique dietary recommendations tailored to Blood Type A+, readers gain insight into how specific foods can positively or negatively impact their health based on their genetic makeup. With a diverse array of recipes ranging from breakfast options to dinner ideas and satisfying snacks, this cookbook empowers individuals to make informed dietary choices that align with their blood type, supporting digestion, energy levels, and overall vitality.

Beyond recipes, this cookbook provides valuable information on meal planning, nutritional needs, and lifestyle recommendations tailored to Blood Type A+ individuals. By embracing a diet rich in plant-based foods, lean proteins, and whole grains while avoiding or minimizing certain foods, readers can embark on a journey towards improved health and well-being. Whether you're new to the Blood Type Diet or seeking fresh culinary inspiration, the Blood Type A+ Diet Cookbook serves as a practical and accessible resource for embracing a nourishing and fulfilling lifestyle in harmony with your blood type.

**PLEASE GO TO THE AMAZON WEBSITE AND LEAVE
A POSITIVE COMMENT AND REVIEW**